COPYCAT RECIPES

The Ultimate Cookbook with Simple and Delicious Recipes for Beginners

TABLE OF CONTENTS

Chapter 1: Benefits of Cooking at Home 5
- Plan for Home Cooking 6
- Get Set for Home Cooking 7
- The Health Benefits 7
  - Social and Emotional Benefits 8
- The Pleasure of Sharing a Homemade Meal 8
- Face Home Cooking Challenges 9

Chapter 2: Taco Bells Recipes 11
1. Taco Bell's Beef Chalupa 11
2. Taco Bell's Enchiritos 13
3. Taco Bell's Double Decker Tacos 16
4. Moe's Southwestern Grill's Steak Quesadilla 18
5. The Mexican Pizza from Taco Bell 20
6. Taco Bell Campfire Chicken 22

Chapter 3: Applebee's Recipes 24
7. Applebee's Triple Chocolate Meltdown 24
8. Three Cheese Chicken Penne from Applebee's 26
9. The Spinach and Artichoke Dip from Applebee's 28
10. Oriental Salad from Applebee's 29
11. Applebee's French Onion Soup 31

Chapter 4: Pasta Recipes 33
12. Pesto Cavatappi from Noodles & Company 33
13. Rattlesnake Pasta from Pizzeria Uno 35
14. Copycat Kung Pao Spaghetti from California Pizza Kitchen .. 37
15. Boston Market Mac n' Cheese 39

16.	Olive Garden's Fettuccine Alfredo	40
17.	Red Lobster's Shrimp Pasta	42
18.	Olive Garden's Steak Gorgonzola	43
19.	Olive Garden Turkey Meatballs over Zucchini Noodles	45
20.	Cheesecake Factory's Pasta Di Vinci	47

Chapter 5: Outback Steakhouse's Recipes 49

21.	Outback Style Steak	49
22.	Longhorn Steakhouse's Mac & Cheese	51
23.	Black Angus Steakhouse's BBQ Baby Back Ribs	52
24.	Outback Steakhouse's Coconut Shrimp	54
25.	Outback's Secret Seasoning Mix for Steaks	55

Chapter 6: Old and Modern Sweet and Savory Snack Recipes 57

26.	Roadhouse Mashed Potatoes	57
27.	Roadhouse Green Beans	59
28.	Roadhouse Cheese Fries	60
29.	Dinner Rolls	61
30.	Texas Red Chili	63
31.	Brined Chicken Bites	65
32.	Blooming' Onion	67
33.	Pepperoni Chips	69
34.	Mac 'n Cheese	70
35.	Red Lobster Lasagna Fritta	72
36.	Red Lobster Spinach Artichoke Dip	74
37.	Red Lobster Fudge Overboard	75
38.	Chocolate Wave	77
39.	Houston's Apple Walnut Cobbler	79

- 40. Papa John's Cinnapie 80
- 41. Olive Garden's Cheese Ziti Al Forno 81
- 42. Olive Garden Meat Overload Pizza 83
- 43. Olive Garden Classic Pepperoni 85
- 44. Olive Garden Meat with Bell Pepper & Mushrooms 86
- 45. Chipotle's Refried Beans 88
- 46. Easy Copycat Monterey's Little Mexico Queso 89
- 47. Fried Keto Cheese with Mushrooms 90
- 48. Mozzarella Cheese Sticks Recipe 91
- 49. Copycat Mac and Cheese with Smoked Gouda Cheese and Pumpkin 92
- 50. Baked Buffalo Meatballs 94

Chapter 7: Chili's 96
- 51. Chili's Black Bean 96
- 52. Chili's Baby Back Ribs 98
- 53. Copycat Chili's Southwest Egg Rolls 100
- 54. Chili's Chicken Enchilada Soup 102
- 55. Cajun Chicken Pasta from Chili's 103

Chapter 1: Benefits of Cooking at Home

Ordering food can be a big problem—time-consuming, costly (an hour for seriously supplying noodles?!), and even tough for your tomb. But of course, it is cheaper, easier, and healthier for your wallet to make alone. Yeah, we're talking about easy, budget-friendly meals you can expect and make in your kitchen in reality. Therefore, it is especially helpful for you if you're one of those who test your food for weight, so you're more conscious of the ingredients. It sounds overwhelming to prepare food for yourself, but you will know that, after all, it's not that difficult. If we say, "Your life will certainly be easier if you know how to make food." However, you must build or arrange your kitchen before you reach the real world of cooking. You need all of them, right out of the kitchen ingredients important foods such as eggs, milk, bread, oil, and lemon, etc. You need all of these tools and cookware. So, we choose the best (and most needed) wineries for wine and dine like a pro, whether we are living and cooking solo for the first time or need an overhaul of our kitchen.

Whether you are a busy parent or yourself, finding the time and energy to prepare home-cooked food can be a daunting challenge. Eating or ordering food at the end of a busy day can be the fastest and easiest choice. Nevertheless, comfort food can significantly affect your mood and health.

The foods produced are normally high in the presence of chemicals, hormones, sugar, salt, excessive fat, and calories that can harm the brain and perception. It makes you feel exhausted, irritable, bloated, and stress, aggravate symptoms of depression, anxiety, and other issues of mental health. It can affect your waistline as well. New research has shown that the total intake of people eating at home is 200 calories a day.

You will ensure that you and your family consume fresh, healthy food by cooking for yourself. It will make you look, feel better, increase stamina, maintain weight and mood, and improve sleep and stress resilience. You are now more aware of what you are putting into your body and of how various foods affect your thoughts and feeling as you cook your food.

It doesn't have to be difficult to cook at home. A portion of food similar to nature has made it the foundation of a balanced diet. It means substituting organic food as many vegetables and safe sources of protein as possible and eating plenty of food. This does not mean spending hours in the kitchen, mixing hundreds of different ingredients, or following intricate recipes with slavishness. Simple foods are also the most delicious so you do not have to be ideal and make every meal at home. Cooking at home will reap benefits just a few days a week.

Often, cooking at home is also a great opportunity for people to spend time with and be a chef. Regardless of your cooking skills and experience, you will learn to make quick and safe meals that help your mental and physical health.

Plan for Home Cooking

It is not a secret that it takes longer to cook at home than to drive or to command. It is important to learn what you must repair before the hour of dinner hits. Begin by making a list of the dinners (or eating), cooking skills, or cooking appreciations. If your mouth is stumped or stuck with the paddle, your mouth and your tummy are sure to groan with a quick search on Pinterest. Give your family some feedback to ensure that their preferences are still on the list.

See your calendar and decide how the meals are going to fit. If you're new to home cooking, start by getting a few meals. If you have a lot to eat, pick the nights when you have some spare time to prepare. When you get more practice, you can pull good meals together faster and with less effort.

For the rest of the month, please make a full menu if you are still used to cooking at home. While I still cook at home, I'm too lazy to take my advice and make a menu occasionally. Having a menu saves you a great deal of work! A ready-to-use will bring your enthusiasm back in the kitchen when you are in a rut or fall off the car. You have a printable weekly meal planner included in the Frugal Fresh Start Workbook. You can get an email when you apply to join the competition if you don't have the workbook.

Get Set for Home Cooking

When you have an idea of what you want to make and want to make it, book a trip into the store to store all the ingredients. See all your recipes and list them well, and you just have to go to the store for one outing. You probably need to stock your pantry with staples because cooking at home is new for you. Try to shop just a week at a time in order not to be distracted. You could prepare a menu and shopping list for longer periods if you are a seasoned Family Chef.

If you're busy with your schedule (or just like saving time), find out what preparation you can do in advance. Can you chop vegetables in the morning or evening before the scheduled meal? Can you prepare a few pot foods and stick them in the freezer over the weekend? When do you get your wife and children involved in the preparations? Preparing something ahead of time makes dinner preparation easier and prevents eating out at the end of a long day.

The Health Benefits

- Preparing healthy foods at home can help your immune system and reduce the risk of heart disease, cancer, high-pressure blood pressure, and diabetes.
- It can help you better manage your health problems; improve how you sleep during the night.
- Cooking healthy food in women can help to reduce PMS and menopause symptoms and increase fertility.
- When you are on a special diet or seek to lose weight, cook food for yourself allows you more control over your ingredients and portion sizes so you can maintain your weight more efficiently, or deal with allergies to food.
- You are less likely to contract a food-borne disease by practicing safe food handling while cooking at home.

- Cooking at home will sharpen your mind, fight cognitive dysfunction, and reduce the risk of Alzheimer's disease.
- It will balance the energy of children and help them become stable and productive adults.

Social and Emotional Benefits

- The quick cooking cycle at home will support and improve your mood and self-esteem.
- This can also be a perfect stress reliever to take time off a busy cooking schedule.
- It can be creatively satisfying to prepare even simple food at home.
- Adopting healthy, homemade meals may enhance your stress, anxiety, and depression resilience and enhance your mood and outlook.
- Cooking and sharing with your family is an ideal way of getting in touch with your loved ones.
- You can expand your social circle to invite friends to join us and reduce stress.
- Eating healthy meals can make your life even happier. You feel happier, both inside and outside of your body, feel healthier.
- Studies have also shown that you are more likely to make healthy decisions when you regularly prepare home-cooked meals while you eat out. In other words, it may become a habit to consume nutritious food.

The Pleasure of Sharing a Homemade Meal

Food brings together people and cooking at home is a great way to bring your family together over the dining table. A homemade meal is everybody's favorite — even smooth teens and picnics, and if you live alone, that's not cooking or eating alone. Sharing food with others is an excellent way to broaden your social network.

- **Become a social experience for meals.** The simple act of talking with a friend or a lover at the table can play a major role in alleviating stress and mood. Join the family and keep up with each other's everyday life. Invite a friend, colleague, or neighbor over if you live alone.

- **Down screens turn down.** Take a break from the television, turn your phone off and avoid other distractions so that the person with whom you are sharing a meal can communicate. You can help prevent emotional overeating by avoiding phones and sharing with others.

- **Cook with others.** Eat with other men. Invite your partner, co-worker, or friend to share the burden of shopping and cooking—for example; one prepares the entrance and another dessert. Cooking with others could be an enjoyable way to deepen your relationships and split the costs for both of you.

Face Home Cooking Challenges

Thinking about your issues at first allowed you to think creatively about how you would overcome your home cooking problems personally. Probably it would be more efficient to develop your solutions rather than answer all your questions, but if you still need some tips, there are a couple of ways to counter the common concerns I mentioned above:

You can cook in your house if you want food or take care of feeding. For example, food and cook seasoning materials have nutrient details on the label. The volume is calculated, and the ingredient is controlled. Also, you will be confident to prepare food by yourself if you want to eat vegetarian food. For certain people to prepare food seriously.

If you order in a high-priced restaurant, you're sure you won't be able to do it because your chef is going to make a kitchen soup. In short, many people today regard eating and exercise as healthy and important. And it's a safe idea to cook at home. Second, it's a smart idea to eat at home to reduce everyday expenses. You have to prepare two or three meals at home, for example, a restaurant for a period. Also, you should use the kitchen to most advantage only to pay rental on the house or the apartment and buy cooking equipment.

If you don't believe me, you should try to find out how much money you can save when you go home to the restaurant. It's a great way to save money you're surprised. Lastly, you can use cooking to improve contact with your family. Home cooking with the other members of your family is a fun activity. You can direct food for your children, for example. You and your kids will help with a healthy relationship.

You can also sit on the TV and watch an entertaining family TV show. Finally, they cook at home and share good or bad moments that occurred at that time. And if you want to develop a family bond, it's a good excuse for your family to start cooking a meal. Ultimately, there are three reasons to endorse the benefit of yourself preparing food. It's a great choice for people who love health care, saving money, and improving family relationships.

Chapter 2: Taco Bells Recipes

1. Taco Bell's Beef Chalupa

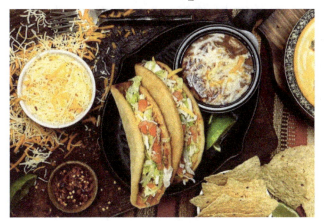

Preparation time: 20 minutes.

Cooking time: 25 minutes.

Servings: 6

Ingredients:

For the fry bread:
- 2(1/2) cups all-purpose flour
- 1 tablespoon baking powder
- ½ teaspoon salt
- 1 tablespoon vegetable shortening
- 1 cup milk

For the filling:
- 1 tablespoon dried onion flakes
- ½ cup water
- 1-pound ground beef

- ¼ cup flour
- 4 teaspoons chili powder
- 1 teaspoon paprika
- 1 teaspoon ground cumin
- 1 teaspoon salt
- ½ teaspoon red pepper flakes

Other ingredients:

- Oil for frying
- Sour cream for serving
- Lettuce for serving
- Grated cheese for serving
- Chopped tomatoes for serving

Directions:

1. Prepare the dough. Combine the flour, baking powder, and salt. Cut in the shortening and mix in the milk. Do not overwork the dough. Cover the bowl and let the dough rest while you prepare the filling.
2. Mix the onion flakes with the water and set them aside to hydrate.
3. In a medium skillet brown the meat, breaking it into small pieces as it cooks. Drain any excess fat. Sprinkle the flour over the beef. Mix and let it cook for a minute or two.
4. Add the onion bits and water. Stir in the spices and mix well. Turn the burner to a minimum and cover the skillet.
5. Turn the fried dough out onto a lightly floured surface and divide it into 8 equal pieces. One at a time, roll them into circles. They should be 8–10 inches across and about a ¼-inch thick. If you want to fold the chalupa, use the rolling pin to press a flat space across the middle of the circle. Heat the oil. Pinch a small ball of

dough (the size of a pea) and drop it in the oil. If the ball immediately floats to the surface, the oil is hot enough.

6. One at a time, lower the dough circles into the oil. Use the tongs to press the dough under the oil, and cook on both sides until golden. Remove them to a plate lined with a paper towel.
7. For folded chalupas, shape them while they're still hot.
8. Add a portion of the meat filling and layer on the desired toppings.

Nutrition:
- **Calories:** 234
- **Carbs:** 2g
- **Fat:** 8.2g
- **Protein:** 12g

2. Taco Bell's Enchiritos

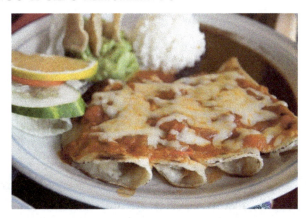

Preparation time: 20 minutes.

Cooking time: 15 minutes.

Servings: 12

Ingredients:

Seasoning:

- 1/4 cup all-purpose flour
- 1 tablespoon chili powder
- 1 teaspoon salt
- ½ teaspoon dried onion flakes
- ½ teaspoon paprika
- ¼ teaspoon onion powder
- 1 dash garlic powder

Tortillas filling:

- 1-pound lean ground beef
- ½ cup water
- 1 (16-ounce) can refried beans
- 12 small flour tortillas
- ½ cup onion, diced
- 1 (16-ounce) can red chili sauce
- 2 cups cheddar cheese, shredded
- Some green onions for serving
- Some sour cream for serving

Directions:

1. Mix all the seasoning ingredients in a bowl.
2. Coat the beef in the seasoning using your hands. Make sure that the beef fully absorbs the flavor from the spices.
3. Brown the seasoned beef in the water over medium heat, for 8 to 10 minutes. Stir the beef occasionally to remove lumps.
4. While the beef is browning, microwave the beans on high for 2 minutes.
5. Wrap the tortillas in a wet towel and microwave for 1 minute.

6. When the beef is done, assemble the tortillas:
    a) Place some beans in the middle of the tortilla.
    b) Place some beef on top, add some onion.
    c) Roll up the tortilla by bringing both ends together in the center.
    d) Place the tortilla in a microwave-safe casserole.
    e) Spread the chili sauce and cheddar cheese on top of the tortilla.
7. Repeat step 5 until the casserole is full.
8. Heat the entire dish in the microwave for 2–3 minutes. The dish is done when the cheese melts.
9. Serve with green onions and sour cream, if desired.

Nutrition:

- **Calories:** 256
- **Carbs:** 12g
- **Fat:** 13.2g
- **Protein:** 12g

3. Taco Bell's Double Decker Tacos

Preparation time: 15 minutes.

Cooking time: 30 minutes.

Servings: 10

Ingredients:

Taco:

- 1 pound ground beef
- 2 tablespoons taco seasoning mix, divided
- 1(16-ounces) can refried beans
- 2/3 cups water
- 12 crisp taco shells
- Sour cream for serving

Guacamole:

- 2 avocados
- 2 tablespoons diced onions
- 1 fresh lime, juiced
- Salt and black pepper to taste
- 12 soft flour tortillas, about 7-inch diameter

Assembling:

- 2 cups shredded cheddar cheese
- 1 cup shredded lettuce
- 1 large tomato, chopped
- ¼ red onion, chopped
- ½ cup sour cream
- Salt and black pepper to taste

Directions:

1. Preheat the oven to 350°F.
2. Cook the beef for 10 to 15 minutes over medium heat, sprinkling it with 3/4 ounce of the taco seasoning. When the beef is brown and crumbly, remove it from the heat and set it aside.
3. Season the refried beans with the remaining taco seasoning mix by placing the beans, water, and seasoning in a small pot and mixing and mashing everything together. Mash the beans and bring the mixture to a simmer.
4. Heat the taco shells in the oven for 3 to 5 minutes.
5. While the taco shells are being heated, make the guacamole by mashing all the guacamole ingredients together.
6. To assemble the tacos, start by covering one side of each flour tortilla with 2 tablespoons of the bean mixture and wrapping the flour tortilla around a taco shell. Then place the following layers inside the taco shell
    a) 2 tablespoons beef.
    b) 2 tablespoons cheese.
    c) Shredded lettuce.
    d) Chopped tomato and onion.
7. Serve with guacamole and sour cream on the side

Nutrition:

- **Calories:** 221
- **Carbs:** 2g
- **Fat:** 8.2g
- **Protein:** 12g

4. Moe's Southwestern Grill's Steak Quesadilla

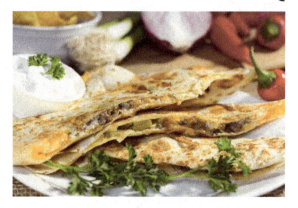

Preparation time: 20 minutes.

Cooking time: 10 minutes.

Servings: 4

Ingredients:

- 4(4-ounce) beef sirloin steaks
- 1 tablespoon olive oil
- 1 small green bell pepper, thinly sliced
- 1 small red bell pepper, thinly sliced
- 1 small yellow bell pepper, thinly sliced
- 1 small yellow onion, thinly sliced
- 1 cup shredded Chihuahua white cheese
- 1 cup shredded American cheese
- 8(8-inch) flour tortillas

For the marinade:

- 3 cloves garlic, minced
- 2 tablespoons chopped parsley
- 3 tablespoons extra virgin olive oil

- 1 teaspoon crushed red chilies
- ½ teaspoon black pepper
- ½ teaspoon salt

Directions:

1. Pound the steaks to an even thickness and place them in a resealable bag. Add the marinade ingredients and turn to coat. Refrigerate for 6 hours or overnight.
2. Heat the olive oil in a skillet and cook the peppers and onion until they are tender-crisp. Remove the vegetables to a bowl and keep them warm.
3. Drain the steaks from the marinade and cook them in the hot skillet for 2–3 minutes on each side until they are cooked to your liking. Rest a few minutes and then slice.
4. Heat a clean skillet over medium heat and place a tortilla in it. Spread some cheese on it, and top with some meat and vegetables. Add more cheese and another tortilla.
5. Cook on both sides until crisp.

Nutrition:

- **Calories:** 241
- **Carbs:** 15g
- **Fat:** 8.2g
- **Protein:** 17g

5. The Mexican Pizza from Taco Bell

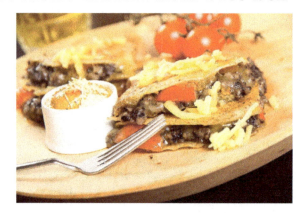

Preparation time: 30 minutes.

Cooking time: 12 minutes.

Servings: 4

Ingredients:

- ½ pound ground beef
- ½ teaspoon salt
- ¼ teaspoon onion, finely chopped
- ¼ teaspoon paprika
- 1(½) teaspoon chili powder
- 2 tablespoons water
- 1 cup vegetable oil
- 8(6-inch) flour tortillas
- 1(16-ounce) can refried beans
- ⅔ cup Picante sauce
- ⅓ cup tomato, finely chopped
- 1 cup cheddar cheese, grated
- 1 cup Colby jack cheese, grated

- ¼ cup green onion, diced
- ¼ cup black olives, chopped

Directions:

1. Preheat oven to 400°F.
2. In a skillet, sauté beef on medium heat. Once brown, drain. Then stir in salt, onions, paprika, chili powder, and water. While continuously stirring, cook for an additional 10 minutes.
3. In a separate skillet, add oil and heat over medium-high. Cook tortilla for about 30 seconds on both sides or until golden brown. Use a fork to pierce any bubbles forming on the tortillas. Transfer onto a plate lined with paper towels.
4. Microwave refried beans on high for about 30 seconds or until warm.
5. To build each pizza, coat ⅓ cup beans on the tortilla followed by ⅓ cup cooked beef. Top with a second tortilla. Cover with 2 tablespoons of Picante sauce, then equal amounts of tomatoes, cheeses, green onions, and olives. This makes a total of 4 pizzas.
6. Place prepared pizzas on a baking sheet. Bake in the oven until cheese is fully melted, about 8 to 12 minutes.
7. Serve.

Nutrition:

- **Calories:** 1218
- **Total fat:** 90g
- **Carbs:** 66g
- **Protein:** 39g
- **Sodium:** 2038mg

6. Taco Bell Campfire Chicken

Preparation time: 19 minutes.

Cooking time: 43 minutes.

Servings: 4

Ingredients:

- 1 tablespoon paprika
- 2 teaspoons onion powder
- 2 teaspoons salt
- 1 teaspoon garlic powder
- 1 teaspoon dried rosemary
- 1 teaspoon black pepper
- 1 teaspoon dried oregano
- 1 whole chicken
- 2 carrots
- 3 red skin potatoes
- 1 ear of corn
- 1 tablespoon olive oil
- 1 tablespoon butter
- 5 sprigs of fresh thyme

Directions:

1. Prepare the oven to 400°F. Blend paprika, onion powder, salt, garlic powder, rosemary, pepper, and oregano. Stir in chicken quarters and 1 tablespoon of the spice mix to a big plastic freezer bag. Seal and chill for 1 hour.

2. Stir in corn, carrots, and potatoes. Drizzle with the olive oil and the remaining spice mix. Toss to coat.
3. Prep a big skillet on high heat. Pour some oil, and once hot, cook chicken pieces until golden brown. Spread 4 pieces of aluminum foil and stir in some carrots, potatoes, corn, and a chicken quarter to each. Drizzle with some butter and thyme.
4. Crease foil in and form pouches by the edges tightly. Bake for 45 minutes.

Nutrition:

- **Calories:** 321
- **Carbohydrates:** 17g
- **Protein:** 26g

Chapter 3: Applebee's Recipes

7. Applebee's Triple Chocolate Meltdown

Preparation time: 25 minutes.

Cooking time: 8 minutes.

Servings: 2–3

Ingredients:

- 4 ounces semisweet chocolate chips
- ½ cup butter
- 2 large whole eggs
- 2 large egg yolks
- ¼ cup sugar, plus more for dusting
- 2 tablespoons of all-purpose flour
- ¼ teaspoon salt

Toppings:

- 4 ounces white chocolate
- 4 ounces semisweet chocolate
- 2 teaspoons vegetable shortening, divided
- 4 scoops of vanilla ice cream

Directions:

1. Preheat the oven to 400°F. Grease muffin pans or ramekins and mud with sugar. Melt chocolate chips with butter over a double saucepan, whisking until smooth.
2. In a separate bowl, whisk together the entire eggs, yolks, and sugar until light and fluffy.

3. Whisk both mixtures together.
4. Gradually add flour and salt, whisking until blended.
5. Distribute evenly into prepared pans and arrange on a baking sheet.
6. Bake until edges are done, and centers are still soft (about 8 minutes).
7. Invert onto the plate.
8. Prepare toppings. Place each sort of chocolate in separate, microwave-safe bowls. Add a teaspoon of shortening to every bowl and cook in the microwave for about 15 seconds and stir. Repeat until smooth.
9. Top the cake pieces with the frozen dessert and drizzle with melted chocolate.

Nutrition:
- **Calories:** 727
- **Total fat:** 31g
- **Carbohydrates:** 107g
- **Protein:** 11g
- **Sodium:** 562mg

8. Three Cheese Chicken Penne from Applebee's

Preparation time: 10 minutes.

Cooking time: 1 hour.

Servings: 4

Ingredients:

- 2 boneless, skinless chicken breasts
- 1 cup Italian salad dressing
- 3 cups penne pasta
- 6 tablespoons olive oil, divided
- 15 ounces Alfredo sauce
- 8 ounces combination mozzarella, Parmesan, and provolone cheeses, grated
- 4 Roma tomatoes, seeded and diced
- 4 tablespoons fresh basil, diced
- 2 cloves garlic, finely chopped
- Shredded parmesan cheese for serving

Directions:

1. Preheat oven to 350°F.
2. In a bowl, add chicken then drizzle with Italian dressing. Mix to coat chicken with dressing fully. Cover using plastic wrap and keep inside the refrigerator overnight but, if you're in a hurry, at least 2 hours is fine.
3. Follow instructions on the package to cook penne pasta. Drain then set aside.
4. Brush 3 tablespoons oil onto grates of the grill then preheat to medium-high heat. Add marinated chicken onto the grill,

discarding the marinade. Cook chicken until both sides are fully cooked and internal temperature measures 165°F. Remove from grill. Set aside until cool enough to handle. Then, cut the chicken into thin slices.

5. In a large bowl, add cooked noodles, Alfredo sauce, and grilled chicken. Mix until combined. Drizzle the remaining oil onto a large casserole pan, then pour the noodle mixture inside. Sprinkle cheeses on top. Bake for about 15–20 minutes or until cheese turns golden and the edges of the mixture begin to bubble. Remove from oven. Mix tomatoes, basil, and garlic in a bowl. Add on top of pasta. Sprinkle parmesan cheese before serving.

Nutrition:

- **Calories:** 1402
- **Fat:** 93g
- **Saturated fat:** 27g
- **Carbs:** 91g
- **Sugar:** 7g
- **Fibers:** 3g
- **Protein:** 62g
- **Sodium:** 5706m

9. The Spinach and Artichoke Dip from Applebee's

Preparation time: 5 minutes.

Cooking time: 30 minutes.

Servings: 10

Ingredients:

- 10-ounce bag spinach, diced
- 14-ounce cans artichoke hearts, diced
- 1 cup Parmesan-Romano cheese mix, grated
- 2 cups mozzarella cheese, grated
- 16 ounces garlic
- 2 tbsp Alfredo sauce
- 8 ounces cream cheese, softened

Directions:

1. Combine all the ingredients in a bowl. Mix well.
2. Transfer into a slow cooker. Set on high and cook for 30 minutes. Serve while hot.

Nutrition:

- **Calories:** 228
- **Fat:** 15g
- **Carbs:** 12g
- **Protein:** 13g
- **Sodium:** 418mg

10. Oriental Salad from Applebee's

Preparation time: 15 minutes.

Cooking time: 5 minutes.

Servings: 6

Ingredients:

- 3 tablespoons of honey
- 1(1/2) tablespoons of rice wine vinegar
- ¼ cup of mayonnaise
- 1 teaspoon Dijon mustard
- 1/8 teaspoon sesame oil
- 3 cups of vegetable oil for frying
- 2 chicken breasts, cut into thin strips
- 1 egg
- 1 cup of milk
- 1 cup of flour
- 1 cup breadcrumbs
- 1 teaspoon salt
- ¼ teaspoon pepper
- 3 cups of romaine lettuce, diced
- ½ cup of red cabbage, diced
- ½ cup of Napa cabbage, diced
- 1 carrot, grated
- ¼ cup of cucumber, diced
- 3 tablespoons of sliced almonds

Directions:

1. To make the dressing, add honey, rice vinegar, mayonnaise, Dijon mustard, and vegetable oil to a blender. Mix until well combined. Store in refrigerator until able to serve.
2. Heat oil in a deep pan over medium-high heat.
3. As the oil warms, whisk together egg and milk in a bowl. In another bowl, add flour, breadcrumbs, salt, and pepper. Mix well.
4. Dredge chicken strips in egg mixture, then in the flour mixture. Confirm the chicken is coated evenly on all sides. Shake off any excess.
5. Deep fry chicken strips for about 3 to 4 minutes until thoroughly cooked and lightly brown. Transfer onto a plate lined with paper towels to empty and funky. Add batches if necessary. Chop strips into small, bite-sized pieces once cool enough to handle.
6. Next, prepare the salad by adding Romaine lettuce, red cabbage, Napa cabbage, carrots, and cucumber to a serving bowl. Top with chicken pieces and almonds. Drizzle the prepared dressing over the top.
7. Serve immediately.

Nutrition:

- **Calories:** 384
- **Total fat:** 13g
- **Saturated fat:** 3g
- **Carbohydrates:** 40g
- **Sugar:** 13g
- **Fibers:** 2g
- **Protein:** 27g
- **Sodium:** 568mg

11. Applebee's French Onion Soup

Preparation time: 25 minutes.

Cooking time: 1 hour and 20 minutes.

Servings: 8

Ingredients:

- 2 tablespoons butter
- 2 tablespoons vegetable oil
- 6 to 7 onions, sliced
- 1 teaspoon salt
- 1(1/2) teaspoon garlic, chopped
- 10 cups beef broth
- 1 tablespoon beef base
- 1 teaspoon black pepper
- 8 slices bread
- 8 teaspoons grated Parmesan cheese
- 8 tablespoons Provolone cheese

Directions:

1. Heat first the butter and oil in a large stockpot over medium heat, then add the sliced onions and salt; sauté the onions until browned. That will take up to half an hour; you want the caramel color of the onions. Frequently remove to prevent burning.
2. Add the chopped garlic when the onions are almost caramelized to the full.
3. Cook the onion and garlic together for about 2 minutes, until the garlic has become fragrant. Add the broth, the base of the beef,

and the black pepper. Taste and if necessary add more salt. Simmer over low heat for 30–45 minutes.

4. Preheat the oven to broil to serve the soup.
5. Ladle soup into 8 individual oven-proof cups, put a slice of bread on top of each, add 1 teaspoon of Parmesan cheese to top each slice, and provolone cheese.
6. Put it under the broiler and cook until the cheese starts browning.
7. Take out in a bowl and enjoy your soup!

Nutrition:
- **Calories:** 300
- **Fat:** 59.8g
- **Carbs:** 35. 6g
- **Protein:** 22.8g
- **Sodium:** 254mg

Chapter 4: Pasta Recipes

12. Pesto Cavatappi from Noodles & Company

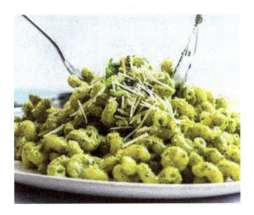

Preparation time: 5 minutes.

Cooking time: 20 minutes.

Servings: 80

Ingredients:

- 4 quarts of water
- 1 tablespoon salt
- 1-pound macaroni pasta
- 1 teaspoon olive oil
- 1 large tomato, finely chopped
- 4-ounce mushrooms, finely chopped
- ¼ cup chicken broth
- ¼ cup dry white wine
- ¼ cup heavy cream
- 1 cup pesto

- 1 cup Parmesan cheese, grated

Directions:

1. Add water and salt to a pot. Bring to a boil. Put in pasta and cook for 10 minutes or until al dente. Drain and set aside.
2. In a pan, heat oil. Sauté tomatoes and mushrooms for 5 minutes. Pour in broth, wine, and cream. Bring to a boil. Reduce heat to medium and simmer for 2 minutes or until the mixture is thick. Stir in pesto and cook for another 2 minutes. Toss in pasta. Mix until fully coated.
3. Transfer onto plates and sprinkle with Parmesan cheese.

Nutrition:

- **Calories:** 637
- **Fat:** 42g
- **Carbs:** 48g
- **Protein:** 19g
- **Sodium:** 1730mg

13. Rattlesnake Pasta from Pizzeria Uno

Preparation time: 5 minutes.

Cooking time: 25 minutes.

Servings: 6

Ingredients:

Pasta:

- 4 quarts of water
- 1-pound penne pasta
- 1 dash of salt

Chicken:

- 2 tablespoons butter
- 2 cloves garlic, finely chopped
- ½ tablespoon Italian seasoning
- 1-pound chicken breast, boneless and skinless, cut into small squares

Sauce:

- 4 tablespoons butter
- 2 cloves garlic, finely chopped
- ¼ cup all-purpose flour
- 1 tablespoon salt
- ¾ teaspoon white pepper
- 2 cups milk
- 1 cup half-and-half
- 3 jalapeno peppers, chopped

Directions:

1. In a pot of boiling water, add salt, and cook pasta according to package instructions. Drain well and set aside.
2. To prepare the chicken, heat butter in a pan. Sauté garlic and Italian seasoning for 1 minute. Add chicken and cook 5–7 minutes or until cooked thoroughly, flipping halfway through. Transfer onto a plate once. Set aside. In the same pan, prepare the sauce. Add butter and heat until melted. Stir in garlic and cook for 30 seconds. Then add flour, salt, and pepper. Cook for 2 more minutes, stirring continuously. Pour in milk and half-and-half. Keep stirring until the sauce turns thick and smooth. Toss in chicken, jalapeno peppers, and pasta. Stir until combined. Serve.

Nutrition:
- **Calories:** 44
- **Fat:** 44g
- **Carbs:** 72g
- **Protein:** 40g
- **Sodium:** 1791mg

14. Copycat Kung Pao Spaghetti from California Pizza Kitchen

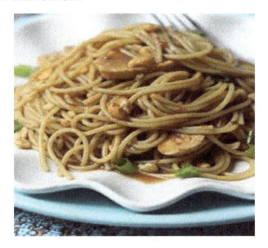

Preparation time: 10 minutes.

Cooking time: 20 minutes.

Servings: 4

Ingredients:

- 1-pound spaghetti
- 2 tablespoons vegetable oil
- 3 chicken breasts, boneless and skinless
- Salt and pepper to taste
- 4 garlic cloves, finely chopped
- ½ cup dry roasted peanuts
- 6 green onions, cut into half-inch pieces
- 10–12 dried bird eyes hot peppers

Sauce:

- ½ cup soy sauce
- ½ cup chicken broth

- ½ cup dry sherry
- 2 tablespoons red chili paste with garlic
- ¼ cup sugar
- 2 tablespoons red wine vinegar
- 2 tablespoons cornstarch
- 1 tablespoon sesame oil

Directions:

1. Follow instructions on the package to cook spaghetti noodles. Drain and set aside.
2. Add oil to a large pan over medium-high heat. Generously season chicken with salt and pepper, then add it to the pan once it is hot. Cook for about 3 to 4 minutes. Turn chicken over and cook for another 3 to 4 minutes. Remove from heat and allow to cool.
3. Mix together all the sauce ingredients in a bowl.
4. Once the chicken is cool enough to handle, chop the chicken into small pieces. Set aside.
5. Return pan to heat. Add garlic and sauté for about 1 minute until aromatic. Pour in the prepared sauce, then stir. Once boiling, lower the heat and allow to simmer for about 1 to 2 minutes or until the liquid thickens. Add pasta, cooked chicken, peanuts, hot peppers, and scallions. Mix well.
6. Serve.

Nutrition:

- **Calories:** 548
- **Fat:** 22g
- **Saturated fat:** 7g
- **Carbs:** 67g
- **Sugars:** 16g

- **Fibers:** 4g
- **Protein:** 15g
- **Sodium:** 2028mg

15. Boston Market Mac n' Cheese

Preparation time: 10 minutes.

Cooking time: 20 minutes.

Servings: 8

Ingredients:

- 8-ounce package spiral pasta
- 2 tablespoons butter
- 2 tablespoons all-purpose flour
- ¾ cups whole milk
- ¼ cup diced processed cheese-like Velveeta™
- ¼ teaspoon dry mustard
- 1 teaspoon salt and pepper to taste

Directions:

1. Cook pasta according to the package instructions. Drain then set aside.
2. To prepare the sauce make the roux with flour and butter over medium-low heat in a large deep skillet. Add milk and whisk until well blended. Add cheese, mustard, salt, and pepper. Keep stirring until smooth.

3. Once pasta is cooked, transfer to a serving bowl. Pour cheese mixture on top. Toss to combine.
4. Serve warm.

Nutrition:
- **Calories:** 319
- **Fat:** 17g
- **Saturated fat:** 10g
- **Carbs:** 28g
- **Sugar:** 7g
- **Fibers:** 1g
- **Protein:** 17g
- **Sodium:** 1134mg

16. Olive Garden's Fettuccine Alfredo

Preparation time: 5 minutes.

Cooking time: 25 minutes.

Servings: 6

Ingredients:
- ½ cup butter, melted
- 2 tablespoons cream cheese
- 1-pint heavy cream
- 1 teaspoon garlic powder
- Some salt
- Some black pepper
- ⅔ cups parmesan cheese, grated

- 1-pound fettuccine, cooked

Directions:

1. Melt the cream cheese in the melted butter over medium heat until soft.
2. Add the heavy cream and season the mixture with garlic powder, salt, and pepper.
3. Reduce the heat to low and allow the mixture to simmer for another 15 to 20 minutes.
4. Remove the mixture from heat and add in the parmesan. Stir everything to melt the cheese.
5. Pour the sauce over the pasta and serve.

Nutrition:

- **Calories:** 767.3
- **Fat:** 52.9g
- **Carbs:** 57.4g
- **Protein:** 17.2g
- **Sodium:** 367mg

17. Red Lobster's Shrimp Pasta

Preparation time: 5 minutes.

Cooking time: 30 minutes.

Servings: 4

Ingredients:

- 8 ounces linguini or spaghetti pasta
- ⅓ cup extra virgin olive oil
- 3 garlic cloves
- 1-pound shrimp, peeled, deveined
- ⅔ cups clam juice or chicken broth
- ⅓ cup white wine
- 1 cup heavy cream
- ½ cup parmesan cheese, freshly grated
- ¼ teaspoon dried basil, crushed
- ¼ teaspoon dried oregano, crushed
- Fresh parsley and parmesan cheese for garnish

Directions:

1. Cook the pasta according to package directions. Simmer the garlic in hot oil over low heat, until tender. Increase the heat from low to medium and add the shrimp. When the shrimp is cooked, transfer it to a separate bowl along with the garlic. Keep the remaining oil in the pan. Pour the clam or chicken broth into the pan and bring to a boil.

2. Add the wine and adjust the heat to medium. Keep cooking the mixture for another 3 minutes. While stirring the mixture, reduce the heat to low and add in the cream and cheese. Keep stirring. When the mixture thickens, return the shrimp to the pan and throw in the remaining ingredients (except the pasta). Place the

pasta in a bowl and pour the sauce over it. Mix everything together and serve. Garnish with parsley and parmesan cheese, if desired.

Nutrition:

- **Calories:** 590
- **Fat:** 26g
- **Carbs:** 54g
- **Protein:** 34g
- **Sodium:** 1500mg

18. Olive Garden's Steak Gorgonzola

Preparation time: 10 minutes.

Cooking time: 1 hour and 30 minutes.

Servings: 6

Ingredients:

Pasta:

- ½ pounds boneless beef top sirloin steaks, cut into ½-inch cubes
- 1-pound fettuccine or linguine, cooked
- 2 tablespoons sun-dried tomatoes, chopped
- 2 tablespoons balsamic vinegar glaze
- Some fresh parsley leaves, chopped

Marinade:

- ½ cups Italian dressing
- 1 tablespoon fresh rosemary, chopped
- 1 tablespoon fresh lemon juice (optional)

Spinach gorgonzola sauce:

- 4 cups baby spinach, trimmed
- 2 cups Alfredo sauce (recipe follows)

- ½ cup green onion, chopped
- 6 tablespoons gorgonzola, crumbled and divided

Directions:

1. Cook the pasta and set it aside. Mix together the marinade ingredients in a sealable container.
2. Marinate the beef in the container for an hour.
3. While the beef is marinating, make the Spinach Gorgonzola sauce. Heat the Alfredo sauce in a saucepan over medium heat. Add spinach and green onions. Let simmer until the spinach wilt. Crumble 4 tablespoons of the Gorgonzola cheese on top of the sauce. Let melt and stir. Set aside the remaining 2 tablespoons of the cheese for garnish. Set aside and cover with the lid to keep warm.
4. When the beef is done marinating, grill each piece depending on your preference.
5. Toss the cooked pasta and the Alfredo sauce in a saucepan and then transfer to a plate.
6. Top the pasta with the beef, and garnish with balsamic glaze, sun-dried tomatoes, crumbled gorgonzola cheese, and parsley leaves.
7. Serve and enjoy.

Nutrition:

- **Calories:** 740.5
- **Fat:** 27.7g
- **Carbs:** 66g
- **Protein:** 54.3g
- **Sodium:** 848.1mg

19. Olive Garden Turkey Meatballs over Zucchini Noodles

Preparation time: 5 minutes.

Cooking time: 15 minutes.

Servings: 4

Ingredients:

- 1 pound ground turkey
- 1/4 cup seasoned dry breadcrumbs
- 1 egg
- 3 tablespoons fresh flat-leaf parsley
- 1(1/2-ounces) Parmesan cheese
- 2 garlic cloves
- 2 tablespoons extra-virgin olive oil
- 1(25-ounces) jar marinara sauce
- 4 medium zucchinis
- 4 ounces Provolone cheese

Directions:

1. Combine each salt and pepper in a bowl with turkey, breadcrumbs, egg, parmesan, 1 garlic clove, and 1/2 teaspoon of parsley.
2. Form into meatballs of 12 (1 ½" to 2"). Heat 1 tablespoon of oil over medium heat in a large skillet.
3. Attach the meatballs and cook for 4 to 6 minutes, turning occasionally, until brown on all sides.
4. Reduce heat in marinara to medium-low and stir gently. Simmer until meatballs are cooked through and the sauce thickened, turning meatballs periodically, 14 to 16 minutes.

5. Meanwhile, over medium to high heat, heat the remaining tablespoon oil in a medium skillet.
6. Add the zucchini and the remaining garlic, and cook for 2 to 3 minutes until tender and moist. Salt and pepper to season.
7. On top, heat the broiler to high with the rack. Sprinkle over meatballs with provolone. Broil for 4 minutes. Serve the meatballs over Parmesan-toped noodles.

Nutrition:

- **Calories:** 246
- **Fat:** 17g
- **Protein:** 9g

20. Cheesecake Factory's Pasta Di Vinci

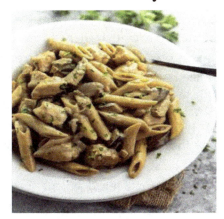

Preparation time: 10 minutes.

Cooking time: 50 minutes.

Servings: 4

Ingredients:

- ½ red onion, chopped
- 1 cup mushrooms, quartered
- 2 teaspoons garlic, chopped
- 1-pound chicken breast, cut into bite-size pieces
- 3 tablespoons butter, divided
- 2 tablespoons flour
- 2 teaspoons salt
- ¼ cup white wine
- 1 cup cream of chicken soup mixed with some milk
- 4 tablespoons heavy cream
- Basil leaves for serving, chopped Parmesan cheese for serving
- 1-pound penne pasta, cooked, drained

Directions:

1. Sauté the onion, mushrooms, and garlic in 1 tablespoon of the butter.
2. When they are tender, remove them from the butter and place them in a bowl. Cook the chicken in the same pan. When the chicken is done, transfer it to the bowl containing the garlic, onions, and mushrooms, and set everything aside.
3. Using the same pan, make a roux using the flour and the remaining butter over low to medium heat. When the roux is ready, mix in the salt, wine, and cream of the chicken mixture. Continue stirring the mixture, making sure that it does not burn. When the mixture thickens, let it simmer for a few more minutes. Mix in the ingredients that you set aside and transfer the cooked pasta to a bowl or plate. Pour the sauce over the pasta, garnish with parmesan cheese and basil, and serve.
4. When the mixture thickens, let it simmer for a few more minutes.

Nutrition:
- **Calories:** 844.9
- **Fat:** 35.8g
- **Carbs:** 96.5g
- **Protein:** 33.9g
- **Sodium:** 1400.2mg

Chapter 5: Outback Steakhouse's Recipes

21. Outback Style Steak

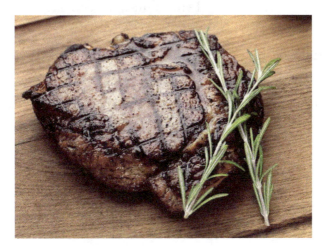

Preparation time: 40 minutes.

Cooking time: 10 minutes.

Servings: 4

Ingredients:

- 4 (6-ounces) sirloin or ribeye steaks
- 2 tablespoons olive oil
- 2 tablespoons old bay seasoning
- 2 tablespoons brown sugar
- 1 teaspoon garlic powder
- 1 teaspoon salt
- ½ teaspoon black pepper
- ½ teaspoon onion powder
- ½ teaspoon ground cumin

Directions:

1. Take the steaks out of the fridge and let them sit at room temperature for about 20 minutes.
2. Combine all the seasonings and mix well.
3. Rub the steaks with oil and some spice mixture, covering all the surfaces. Let the steaks sit for 20–30 minutes.
4. Meanwhile, heat your grill to medium-high.
5. Cook the steaks for about 5 minutes on each side for medium-rare (or to an internal temperature of 130°F). Let them sit for 5 minutes before serving.

Nutrition:

- **Calories:** 254
- **Total fat:** 13g
- **Carbs:** 56g
- **Protein:** 45g
- **Fiber:** 3g

22. Longhorn Steakhouse's Mac & Cheese

Preparation time: 20 minutes.

Cooking time: 20 minutes.

Servings: 10

Ingredients:

- 1-pound Cavatappi pasta, cooked
- 2 tablespoons butter
- 2 tablespoons flour
- 2 cups half-and-half
- 2 ounces gruyere cheese, shredded
- 8 ounces white cheddar, shredded
- 2 tablespoons parmesan cheese, shredded
- 4 ounces Fontina cheese, shredded
- 1 teaspoon smoked paprika
- 4 pieces bacon, crispy, crumbled
- ½ cup panko bread crumbs

Directions:

1. Make a roux by cooking the melted butter and flour over medium heat.
2. When the roux is cooked, add in the half-and-half ½ cup at a time, adding more as the sauce thickens.
3. Slowly add the rest of the ingredients (except the pasta) one at a time, really allowing each ingredient to incorporate itself into the sauce. Continue stirring the mixture until everything is heated.
4. Place the pasta in a greased 13×9 baking pan or 6 individual baking dishes and pour the sauce over it. Sprinkle the bacon and panko bread crumbs over the top of the pasta.

5. Bake the pasta in an oven preheated to 350°F for 20–25 minutes, or until breadcrumbs start to become golden brown.
6. Let the pasta cool and serve.

Nutrition:

- **Calories:** 610
- **Fat:** 37g
- **Carbs:** 43g
- **Protein:** 26g ; **Sodium:** 1210mg

23.   Black Angus Steakhouse's BBQ Baby Back Ribs

Preparation time: 30 minutes.

Cooking time: 6 to 8 hours.

Servings: 1

Ingredients:

- 1 rack of pork ribs
- Your favorite barbecue sauces
- Onion powder to taste
- Garlic powder to taste

Marinade:

- 2 tablespoons kosher salt
- 2 tablespoons paprika
- 4 tablespoons granulated garlic
- 1 tablespoon onion powder
- 1 teaspoon cumin seeds

- 1 teaspoon Durfee Ancho pepper
- 2 teaspoons dry mustard
- 2 teaspoons black pepper

Rib mop:

- 1 cup red wine vinegar
- 1 tablespoon garlic
- 1 cup water
- 3 tablespoons soy sauce

Directions:

1. Mix all the marinade ingredients together. Rub the marinade all over the ribs to soak them in flavor.
2. Barbecue the meat over indirect heat at 250°F to 300°F for 3 to 4 hours. Add soaked fruitwood to the coals for additional aroma. Make sure that the temperature remains at 250°F to 300°F for the entire cooking duration. While the meat is cooking, mix together the rib mop ingredients in a bowl.
3. After three to four hours, transfer the meat to an aluminum pan and brush both sides with the rib mop.
4. Cook the ribs for another hour and then remove them from heat and mop them again. Continue cooking the ribs for another 3 to 4 hours, basting them with the mop and some barbecue sauce every hour. When the ribs are done barbecuing, sprinkle them with onion and garlic powder before wrapping them in aluminum foil. Let the ribs rest for 30 minutes.
5. Situate the ribs to a plate and serve.

Nutrition:

- **Calories:** 1500
- **Total Fat:** 30g
- **Protein:** 14

24. Outback Steakhouse's Coconut Shrimp

Preparation time: 10 minutes.

Cooking time: 14 minutes.

Servings: 4

Ingredients:

- 1 pound medium shrimp, tail removed, peeled, deveined, and cooked
- ½ cup pork rind
- 1 teaspoon salt
- ½ cup shredded coconut, unsweetened
- ½ teaspoon ground black pepper
- ¼ cup coconut milk, unsweetened

Directions:

1. Take a shallow pan, place it over low heat and when hot, add coconut and cook for 3 to 4 minutes until golden brown.
2. Take a shallow dish, then pour within the milk.
3. Take a separate shallow dish, place coconut and pork rind in it, and then stir until mixed.
4. Pat dry the shrimp with paper towels, then dip each shrimp into milk and dredge within the pork-coconut mixture until evenly coated.
5. Plugin the air fryer, insert a greased fryer basket, set it 400°F, and let it preheat for 400°F.
6. Then add shrimps during a single layer into the fryer basket, then fry for 7 minutes, shaking halfway.
7. When done, transfer fried shrimps to a plate and repeat with the remaining shrimps.
8. Add black pepper and salt to the shrimps, then serve.

Nutrition:

- **Calories:** 335
- **Fats:** 15.6g
- **Protein:** 46.1g
- **Net carb:** 0.9g
- **Fiber:** 1.7g

25. Outback's Secret Seasoning Mix for Steaks

Preparation time: 5 minutes.

Cooking time: 10 minutes.

Servings: 3

Ingredients:

Seasoning:

- 4–6 teaspoons salt
- 4 teaspoons paprika
- 2 teaspoons ground black pepper
- 1 teaspoon onion powder
- 1 teaspoon garlic powder
- 1 teaspoon cayenne pepper
- ½ teaspoon coriander
- ½ teaspoon turmeric

Directions:

1. Blend all the seasoning ingredients in a bowl. Rub the spice blend into the meat on all sides and let rest for 15–20 minutes before cooking.

Nutrition:
- **Calories:** 16.4
- **Total fat:** 0.5g
- **Carbohydrates:** 3.5g

Chapter 6: Old and Modern Sweet and Savory Snack Recipes

26.   Roadhouse Mashed Potatoes

Preparation time: 20 minutes.

Cooking time: 30 minutes.

Servings: 6

Ingredients:

- ¼ cup Parmesan cheese, grated
- 1 whole garlic bulb
- ¼ cup sour cream
- 4 medium potatoes, peeled & quartered
- ¼ cup each of softened butter & 2% milk
- 1 teaspoon plus
- 1 tablespoon olive oil, divided
- ¼ teaspoon pepper
- 1 medium white onion, chopped
- ½ teaspoon salt

Directions:

1. Preheat the oven to 425°F. Cut off the papery outer skin from the garlic bulb; ensure that you don't separate the cloves or peel them. Remove the top from the garlic bulb, exposing individual cloves. Brush cut cloves with approximately 1 teaspoon of oil, then wrap in foil. Bake in the preheated oven for 30 to 35 minutes until cloves are soft.

2. Meanwhile, cook the leftover oil over low heat. Once done, add & cook the chopped onion for 15 to 20 minutes, until golden brown, stirring now and then. Transfer to a food processor. Process on high until blended well; set aside.

3. Put the potatoes in a large saucepan and cover them with water. Bring to a boil. Once done, decrease the heat; cook for 15 to 20 minutes, until tender, uncovered. Drain and return to the pan. Squeeze the softened garlic over the potatoes; add butter, cheese, sour cream, milk, onion, pepper, and salt. Beat until mashed. Serve and enjoy.

Nutrition:
- **Calories:** 220
- **Total fats:** 15g
- **Protein:** 3g

27. Roadhouse Green Beans

Preparation time: 10 minutes.

Cooking time: 20 minutes.

Servings: 8

Ingredients:

- 2 cans green beans (16 ounces), drained
- 1 tablespoon sugar
- 4 ounces bacon, diced (raw) or 4 ounces ham (cooked)
- 2 cups water
- 4 ounces onions, diced
- ½ teaspoon pepper

Directions:

1. Thoroughly drain green beans using a colander; set aside. Combine pepper with sugar & water until incorporated well; set aside. Preheat your cooking pan over medium-high heat.
2. Dice the cooked ham into equal size pieces using a cutting board and a knife. Place the diced onions and ham into the preheated cooking pan. Continue to stir the onions and ham using the large spoon until the onions are tender and the ham is lightly brown.
3. Once done, add the beans and liquid mixture. Using the rubber spatula, give the mixture a good stir until incorporated well. Let the mixture boil, then lower the heat to simmer. Serve the beans as soon as you are ready and enjoy.

Nutrition:

- **Calories:** 221
- **Total fats:** 16g
- **Protein:** 4g

28. Roadhouse Cheese Fries

Preparation time: 20 minutes.

Cooking time: 30 minutes.

Servings: 4

Ingredients:

- 6–8 slices bacon, enough to make ½ cup once cooked
- 4 cups steak-style French fries, frozen
- ¼ teaspoon onion powder
- 2 cups sharp cheddar cheese, grated
- Oil for frying
- ¼ teaspoon each of garlic salt & seasoning salt

Directions:

1. Preheat your oven to 450°F. Cook the bacon over medium-high heat in a medium-sized frying pan. Take out the bacon when crisp & place it on a paper towel to drain.

2. Pour the bacon grease into a bowl & let it slightly cool. Add onion powder, seasoned salt, and garlic salt to the grease; combine well and set aside. Assemble the fries on a greased baking sheet & bake in the preheated oven until turn slightly golden, for 10 to 15 minutes.

3. Set your oven to broil. Brush the bacon oil with the seasoning mix onto each fry. Place fries in an oven-safe bowl. Spread the cheddar cheese on top of the fries. Crumble bacon slices and then sprinkle on top of the cheese.

4. Place the dish in the oven until the cheese is bubbly, for 3 to 5 minutes. Remove from the oven & let sit for a couple of minutes, then serve.

Nutrition:

- **Calories:** 188
- **Total fats:** 11g
- **Protein:** 4g

29. Dinner Rolls

Preparation time: 1 hour.

Cooking time: 15 minutes.

Servings: 4

Ingredients:

For rolls:

- 2(¼) teaspoon or 1 packet active dry yeast
- 1 large egg, at room temperature
- 1 ¼ cup milk
- 4 tablespoons melted butter, separated
- ¼ cup honey
- 4 cups flour
- 1 teaspoon salt

For Texas roadhouse butter:

- ¼ cup powdered sugar
- 1 stick salted butter, at room temperature for an hour
- ¾ teaspoon cinnamon
- 1(½) tablespoons honey

Directions:

For Texas roadhouse butter

1. Using an electric mixer, combine the entire Roadhouse butter ingredients together until smooth & creamy. Refrigerate until ready to use.

For rolls:

2. Bring the milk to a boil over moderate heat. Once done, remove the pan from heat & set it aside at room temperature until lukewarm.

3. Now, combine the milk with honey & yeast in a small bowl until combined well. Let sit for a couple of minutes. Combine 2 cups of flour with milk mixture, egg & 3 tablespoons of butter in a large bowl. Slowly mix until smooth. Slowly add the leftover flour & continue to mix until the dough-like consistency is achieved.

4. Add salt & continue to mix for 6 to 8 more minutes. Drop the dough onto a floured surface; knead for a couple of minutes more. Grease the large bowl with the cooking spray & drop the dough inside. Using plastic wrap, cover the bowl & let rise in a warm place for an hour.

5. Coat 2 cookie sheets lightly with the vegetable oil. Punch the dough down & roll it out on a flat, floured surface until it's approximately ½" thick. Fold it in half & gently seal. Evenly cut the dough into 24 squares & arrange them on the prepared cookie sheets. Using a plastic wrap, cover & let them rise until almost doubled in size, for 35 to 40 minutes.

6. Preheat your oven to 350°F in advance & bake until the top is a light golden brown, for 12 to 15 minutes. Heat the leftover tablespoon of butter until melted and then brush the top of the rolls.

7. Serve with Texas roadhouse butter and enjoy.

Nutrition:

- **Calories:** 210
- **Total fats:** 14g; **Protein:** 5g

30. Texas Red Chili

Preparation time: 2 minutes.

Cooking time: 5 minutes.

Servings: 4

Ingredients:

- 2(½) pounds boneless beef chuck, well-trimmed & cut into ¾" cubes
- 1(½) teaspoons ground cumin seed
- 2 ounces papilla chilis
- ⅓ cup onion, finely chopped
- 3 large garlic cloves, minced
- 2(¼) cups water, plus more as needed
- Sour cream for serving
- 1 tablespoon firmly packed dark brown sugar, plus more as needed
- 2 tablespoons masa harina (corn tortilla flour)
- 1(½) tablespoon distilled white vinegar, plus more as needed
- 2 cups canned low-sodium beef broth or beef stock, plus more as required
- Lime wedges for serving
- ½ teaspoon freshly ground black pepper
- 5 tablespoons vegetable oil, lard or rendered beef suet
- Kosher salt to taste

Directions:

1. Over medium-low heat in a straight-sided large skillet; gently toast the chilies for 2 to 3 minutes per side, until fragrant. Keep an eye

on them and don't let them burn. Place the chilies in a large bowl & cover them with very hot water; let soak for 15 to 45 minutes, until soft, turning a couple of times during the soaking process.

2. Drain the chiles; split them & remove the seeds and stems. Place the chilies in a blender & then add the black pepper, cumin, ¼ cup water, and 1 tablespoon salt. Purée the mixture until a smooth, slightly fluid paste forms; feel free to add more water as required and scrape down the sides of your blender jar occasionally. Set aside until ready to use.

3. Place the skillet over medium-high heat again & heat 2 tablespoons of lard until melted. When it starts to smoke, swirl to coat the bottom of your skillet & add half of the beef. Lightly brown on at least two sides, for 2 to 3 minutes on each side. If the meat threatens to burn, immediately decrease the heat. Transfer to a bowl & repeat with 2 more tablespoons of lard & the leftover beef. Reserve.

4. Let the skillet cool slightly & place it over medium-low heat. Heat the leftover lard in the same skillet. Once melted, immediately add the garlic and onion; gently cook for 3 to 4 minutes, stirring now and then. Add the stock & the leftover water; slowly whisk in the masa harina to avoid lumps. Stir in the reserved chili paste, scraping the bottom of your skillet using a spatula to loosen any browned bits. Place the reserved beef (along with any accumulated juices) & bring to a simmer over high heat. Once done, decrease the heat to maintain the barest possible simmer & continue to cook for 2 hours, until 1 ½ to 2 cups of thickened but still liquid sauce surrounds the cubes of meat & the meat is tender but still somewhat firm, stirring occasionally.

5. Thoroughly stir in the vinegar & brown sugar; add more salt to taste; let simmer gently for 10 more minutes. Switch it off and set it aside for 30 minutes. If the mixture appears to be too dry, feel free to stir in the additional water or broth. Alternatively, let it simmer a couple of more minutes if the mixture appears to be a

little loose & wet. Alter the balance of flavors with a bit of additional vinegar, sugar, or salt, if desired.

6. Gently reheat & serve in separate bowls with a dollop of sour cream on top & a fresh lime wedge on the side.

Nutrition:
- **Calories:** 218
- **Total fats:** 13g
- **Protein:** 4g

31. Brined Chicken Bites

Preparation time: 10 minutes.

Cooking time: 20 minutes.

Servings: 4

Ingredients:
- 1 pound chicken breast
- ½ teaspoon salt
- 2 cups pickle juice
- Avocado oil, as needed for frying

For the coating:
- 1 tablespoon baking powder
- ½ teaspoon garlic powder
- ½ teaspoon salt
- 1 tablespoon erythritol sweetener
- ½ teaspoon ground black pepper
- ½ teaspoon paprika
- ½ cup whey protein powder

Directions:

1. Cut the chicken into 1-inch pieces, place them in a large plastic bag, add salt, pour in pickle juice, and then seal the bag.
2. Turn it upside down to coat the chicken pieces and then let marinate for a minimum of 30 minutes in the refrigerator.
3. Then remove chicken from the refrigerator, let it rest at room temperature for 25 minutes, drain it well, and pat dry with paper towels.
4. Cook the chicken and for this, take a large pot, place it over medium-low heat, pour in oil until the pot has half-full, and then bring it to 350°F.
5. Meanwhile, prepare the coating and for this, take a medium bowl, place all of its ingredients in it and then stir until mixed.
6. Dredge a chicken piece into the coating mixture until thoroughly covered, arrange it onto a baking sheet lined with parchment paper and repeat with the remaining pieces.
7. Drop the prepared chicken pieces into the oil, fry for 6 minutes until thoroughly cooked, and then transfer to a plate lined with paper towels. Repeat with the remaining chicken pieces and then serve.

Nutrition:

- **Calories:** 284
- **Fats:** 17g
- **Protein:** 34g
- **Carb:** 1g

32. Blooming' Onion

Preparation time: 15 minutes.

Cooking time: 5 minutes.

Servings: 4

Ingredients:

- 1 large sweet onion
- ½ cup coconut flour
- ½ tablespoon seasoning salt
- ½ teaspoon ground black pepper
- ½ teaspoon cayenne
- ½ tablespoon paprika
- 4 tablespoons heavy whipping cream
- 4 eggs
- 1 cup pork rind
- Avocado oil, as needed for frying

Directions:

1. Prepare the onion and for this, remove ¼ top off the onion, flip it cut-side-down and then cut it into quarters in such a way that there is only ¼-inch space from the onion nub. Cut the quarters into eights and then cut them into sixteenths.

2. Sprinkle coconut flour generously over the onion until each petal and the bottom of the onion have coated.

3. Prepare the egg wash and for this, take a medium bowl, crack the eggs in it, whisk in the cream until blended, and then spoon half of this mixture over the onion until each petal and the bottom of the onion have coated.

4. Take a separate medium bowl, place pork rind in it, add all the seasonings, stir until mixed, and then coat onion inside out with this mixture.

5. Repeat by pouring the remaining egg wash over the onion and dredge again into pork rind mixture.

6. Transfer onion onto a plate and then freeze it for 1 hour.

7. When ready to cook, take a large pot, place it over medium-high heat, fill it two-thirds with oil, and bring it to 300°F temperature.

8. Then lower the frozen onion into the oil, petal-side-down, and cook for 1 month, switch heat to medium-low level, flip the onion and fry it for 3 minutes.

9. Transfer onion to a plate lined with paper towels and let it rest for 5 minutes.

10. Serve the onion with dipping sauce.

Nutrition:
- **Calories:** 514
- **Fats:** 30.3g
- **Proteins:** 47.2g
- **Carbs:** 10g

33. Pepperoni Chips

Preparation time: 5 minutes.

Cooking time: 8 minutes.

Servings: 2

Ingredients:

- 30 pepperoni slices

Directions:

1. Switch on the oven, set it to 400°F, then set the baking rack in the middle and let it preheat. Meanwhile, take a sheet pan or two-lines with parchment paper, and then spread pepperoni slices o with some spacing between each slice.
2. Bake the pepperoni slices for 4 minutes, then pat dry them with paper towels and then continue baking them for 4 minutes until nicely golden brown.
3. When done, drain the pepperoni slices on paper towels and then serve.

Nutrition:

- **Calories:** 150
- **Fats:** 14g
- **Protein:** 5g
- **Carbs:** 1g

34. Mac 'n Cheese

Preparation time: 20 minutes.

Cooking time: 20 minutes.

Servings: 12

Ingredients:

- 4 or 5 tablespoons flour
- ¼ teaspoon each of ground white pepper & red-hot sauce
- 2 or 3 cups half and half
- ½ teaspoon creole seasoning or essence
- 4 tablespoons butter, plus 2 tablespoons, plus 1 tablespoon
- 8(½) ounces Parmigiano-Reggiano parmesan cheese, grated
- ¼ cup breadcrumbs, fresh
- 1-pound elbow macaroni
- ½ teaspoon garlic, minced
- 4 ounces each of cheddar cheese, gruyere cheese & Fontina cheese, grated
- ¾ teaspoons salt

Directions:

1. Over low heat in a heavy, medium saucepan; heat 3 or 4 tablespoons of butter until melted. Add the flour; turn to combine & cook for 3 to 4 minutes, stirring constantly. Increase the heat to medium; slowly whisk in the half and half. Cook for 4 to 5 minutes, until thickened, stirring frequently. Remove from the heat and season with 4 ounces of the grated parmesan, hot sauce, pepper, and salt. Give the ingredients a good stir until cheese is completely melted & sauce is smooth. Cover & set aside.
2. Preheat your oven to 340°F in advance.

3. Fill a pot with water; bring it to a boil. Add the macaroni and salt to taste, stir well. Bring it to a boil again. Once done, decrease the heat to a low boil & continue to cook until macaroni is al dente, for 5 minutes. Drain the macaroni in a colander and put the macaroni in the pot. Add 2 tablespoons of butter and garlic; stir until everything blends. Add the bechamel sauce; stir until combined well. Set aside until ready to use.

4. Grease a 3-quart casserole or baking dish using the leftover butter & set aside. Combine the leftover parmesan cheese together with cheddar, Fontina, and gruyere cheeses in a large bowl; toss until combined well.

5. Place 1/3 of the macaroni in the prepared baking dish. Add 1/3 of the mixed cheeses on top. Top with another third of the macaroni and another third of the mixture of cheese. Repeat with the leftover macaroni & cheese mixture. Combine the breadcrumbs together with leftover grated parmesan & the Essence in a small bowl; toss until combined well. Sprinkle this on top of the macaroni and cheese.

6. Bake until the macaroni & cheese is bubbly and hot, and the top is golden brown, for 40 to 45 minutes. Remove from oven & let sit for 5 minutes before serving.

Nutrition:

- **Calories:** 143
- **Fats:** 11g
- **Protein:** 8g
- **Carbs:** 4g

35. Red Lobster Lasagna Fritta

Preparation time: 10 minutes.

Cooking time: 10 minutes.

Servings: 4–6

Ingredients:

- 2/3 + ¼ cups milk (divided)
- 1 cup grated parmesan cheese, plus some more for serving
- 3/4 cups feta cheese
- 1/4 teaspoon white pepper
- 1 tablespoon butter
- 7 lasagna noodles
- 1 egg
- ½ lb. Breadcrumbs
- Oil for frying
- 2 tablespoons marinara sauce
- Alfredo sauce for serving

Directions:

1. Place the butter, white pepper, 2/3 cup milk, parmesan, and feta cheese in a pot. Stir and boil.
2. Prepare lasagna noodles according to instructions on the package.
3. Spread a thin layer of the cheese and milk mixture on each noodle. Fold into 2-inch pieces and place something heavy on top to keep them folded. Place in the freezer for at least 1 hour, then cut each noodle in half lengthwise.
4. In a small bowl, mix the ¼ cup milk and egg. In another bowl, place breadcrumbs.

5. Dip each piece into the egg wash, then the breadcrumbs. Fry the noodles at 350°F for 4 minutes.

6. Serve by spreading some Alfredo sauce at the bottom of the plate, placing the lasagna on top, and then drizzling with marinara sauce. Garnish with a sprinkle of grated parmesan cheese

Nutrition:

- **Calories** 218
- **Total fat** 15g
- **Carbs** 12g
- **Protein** 13g
- **Sodium** 418mg

36. Red Lobster Spinach Artichoke Dip

Preparation time: 15 minutes.

Cooking time: 10 minutes.

Servings: 4

Ingredients:

- 3 tablespoons butter
- 3 tablespoons flour
- 1(1/2) cup milk
- ½ teaspoon salt
- ¼ teaspoon black pepper
- 5 ounces spinach, frozen and chopped
- ¼ cup artichokes, diced (I like to use marinated)
- ½ teaspoon garlic, chopped
- ½ cup parmesan, shredded
- ½ cup mozzarella, shredded
- 1 tablespoon Asiago cheese, shredded
- 1 tablespoon Romano cheese, shredded
- 2 tablespoons cream cheese
- ¼ cup mozzarella cheese (for topping)

Directions:

1. Melt butter over medium heat in a saucepan. Add flour and cook for about 1–2 minutes. Add milk and stir until thick.
2. Season with salt and pepper to taste. Add spinach, diced artichokes, garlic, cheeses, and cream cheese to the pan. Stir until warmed.

3. Pour into a small baking dish. Sprinkle mozzarella cheese on top and place under the broiler. Broil until the top begins browning.

Nutrition:
- **Calories** 238
- **Total fat** 15g
- **Carbs** 12g
- **Protein** 13g
- **Sodium** 418mg

37. Red Lobster Fudge Overboard

Preparation time: 10 minutes.

Cooking time: 15 minutes.

Servings: 4

Ingredients

For the pecan brownies:
- 13 x 9 family size package of brownie mix
- Olive oil required per the package directions
- Egg (required as per the number mentioned on the package)
- ½ cup pecans, chopped

For the chocolate sauce:
- ½ cup butter
- 4 unsweetened chocolate squares
- 1 can of evaporated milk (12 ounces)
- 3 cups sugar
- ½ teaspoon salt

For the whipped cream:

- 1 can of canned whip whipped cream

Directions:

For the pecan brownies:

1. Follow the directions mentioned on the brownie mix and then add approximately ½ cup of the chopped pecans. Pour the prepared mixture into a large pan. Bake as per the directions mentioned on the package.

For the chocolate sauce:

2. Over low heat in a large, heavy saucepan; melt the butter & chocolate, stirring constantly. Slowly add the sugar, alternately with the evaporated milk, starting & ending with sugar; continue to stir until smooth, for 5 minutes, over medium heat. Stir in the salt.

For the whipped cream:

3. Microwave the chocolate sauce and brownie in separate dishes; ensure it's hot. After microwaving the brownie, place a scoop of ice cream on top. Drizzle the hot chocolate sauce on top of the ice cream and then top with the whipped cream.

Nutrition:

- **Calories:** 169
- **Fat:** 10g
- **Carbs:** 19g
- **Protein:** 33g

38. Chocolate Wave

Preparation time: 25 minutes.

Cooking time: 5 hours and 15 minutes.

Servings: 6

Ingredients:

- 4 organic eggs, large
- 1 cup sugar
- 2(½) teaspoons cornstarch
- ¾ cup butter
- 4 egg yolks
- 1 cup semisweet chocolate chips
- 1(½) teaspoon Grand Marnier

For white-chocolate truffle:

- 3 tablespoons heavy cream
- 6 ounces white chocolate
- 2 tablespoons Grand Marnier
- 3 tablespoons softened butter

Directions:

1. Over medium-low heat in a double boiler; melt the butter. Add in the chocolate chips; continue to heat until the mixture is completely melted.
2. Combine cornstarch and sugar in a large-sized mixing bowl. Add the chocolate mixture into the sugar mixture; beat well.
3. Combine four yolks with four eggs & Grand Marnier in a separate bowl. Add this to the chocolate mixture; continue to beat until mixed well. Cover & let chill overnight.

4. **For truffle:** Over low heat in a double boiler; melt the white chocolate with heavy cream. Add Grand Marnier and butter; give the ingredients a good stir until completely smooth. Chill for overnight.

5. Lightly coat 5-ounce ramekins with butter & then dust with flour, filling approximately 1/3 of the chilled chocolate mixture. Add a rounded tablespoon of the truffle mixture. Fill to the top with the chocolate mixture.

6. Bake for 15 minutes at 450°F. Let the cakes sit for 15 to 20 minutes before inverting. Run a knife around the edges to loosen. Serve with raspberries, chocolate sauce, and/or ice cream.

Nutrition:

- **Calories:** 302
- **Fat:** 22g
- **Carbs:** 28g
- **Protein:** 35g

39. Houston's Apple Walnut Cobbler

Preparation time: 15 minutes.

Cooking time: 30 minutes.

Servings: 6

Ingredients:

- 3 large Granny Smith apples, peeled and diced
- 1(½) cup walnuts, coarsely chopped
- 1 cup all-purpose flour
- 1 cup brown sugar
- 1 teaspoon cinnamon
- Pinch of nutmeg
- 1 large egg
- ½ cup (1 stick) butter, melted
- Vanilla ice cream
- Caramel sauce for drizzling

Directions:

1. Preheat oven to 350°F. Lightly grease an 8-inch square baking dish. Spread diced apple over the bottom of the baking dish.
2. Sprinkle with walnuts. In a bowl, mix together flour, sugar, cinnamon, nutmeg, and egg to make a coarse-textured mixture.
3. Sprinkle over the apple-walnut layer. Pour melted butter over the whole mixture. Bake until fragrant and crumb top is browned (about 30 minutes). Serve warm topped with scoops of vanilla ice cream.
4. Drizzle with caramel sauce.

Nutrition:

- **Calories:** 611

- **Fat:** 36g
- **Carbs:** 69g
- **Protein:** 8g

40. Papa John's Cinnapie

Preparation time: 5 minutes.

Cooking time: 12 minutes.

Servings: 12

Ingredients:

- 1 whole pizza dough
- 1 tablespoon melted butter
- 2 tablespoons cinnamon, or to taste

Topping:

- ¾ cups flour
- ½ cup white sugar
- 1/3 cup brown sugar
- 2 tablespoons oil
- 2 tablespoons shortening

Icing:

- 1(½) cup powdered sugar
- 3 tablespoons milk
- ¾ teaspoons vanilla

Directions:

1. Preheat oven to 460°F. Grease or spray a pizza pan or baking sheet.

2. Brush the dough evenly with melted butter. Sprinkle with cinnamon. Place the ingredients for the topping in a bowl and toss together with a fork.

3. Sprinkle topping over the dough. Bake until fragrant and lightly browned at the edges (about 10–12 minutes). Mix the icing ingredients together in a bowl. If too thick, gradually add in a little more milk. Drizzle icing over warm pizza.

Nutrition:
- **Calories:** 560
- **Carbs:** 90g
- **Fat:** 19g
- **Protein:** 8g

41. Olive Garden's Cheese Ziti Al Forno

Preparation time: 10 minutes.

Cooking time: 35 minutes.

Servings: 8

Ingredients:
- 1 pound ziti
- 4 tablespoons butter
- 2 cloves garlic
- 4 tablespoons all-purpose flour
- 2 cups half & half
- A dash of black pepper
- Kosher salt (as desired)
- 3 cups marinara

- 1 cup grated parmesan, divided
- 2 cups shredded mozzarella, divided

Other shredded cheese:

- ½ cup Fontina
- ½ cup Romano
- ½ cup ricotta
- ½ cup panko breadcrumbs

The garnish:

- Fresh parsley

Directions:

1. Warm the oven to reach 375°F.
2. Spritz the casserole dish with cooking oil spray. Prepare a large pot of boiling - salted water to cook the ziti until al dente. Drain and set it to the side.
3. Mince the garlic. Shred/grate the cheese and chop the parsley.
4. Make the Alfredo. Heat the skillet using the medium temperature setting to melt the butter. Toss in the garlic to sauté for about half a minute. Whisk in flour and simmer until the sauce is bubbling (1–2 minutes).
5. Whisk in the half-and-half and simmer. Stir in ½ cup parmesan, pepper, and salt. Cook it until the sauce thickens (2–3 minutes). Stir in the marinara, one cup of mozzarella, Romano, Fontina, and ricotta. Fold in the pasta. Dump it into the casserole dish.
6. Combine ½ cup of the parmesan and the breadcrumbs. Sprinkle it over the top of the dish. Set the timer and bake until browned as desired and bubbly (30 minutes). Garnish with parsley and serve.

Nutrition:

- **Calories:** 272

- **Fat:** 20g
- **Carbs:** 25g
- **Protein:** 23g

42. Olive Garden Meat Overload Pizza

Preparation time: 25 minutes.

Cooking time: 25 minutes.

Servings: 8

Ingredients:

- 1 thin pizza crust, or crust of choice
- 1/2-3/4 cups marinara sauce
- 2 tablespoons olive oil
- 1(1/2)–2 pounds assorted meat like ground beef, pepperoni, Italian sausage, breakfast sausage, ham (chopped), and bacon
- Salt and pepper to taste
- 2 cups mozzarella cheese

Directions:

1. Heat oven to 425°F.
2. Cook bacon until crisp. Cool slightly and then crumble.
3. Cook sausages in a little oil over medium heat to brown. Drain over paper towels.
4. Season ground beef with salt and pepper and sauté until browned. Drain.
5. Spread sauce over dough.

6. Sprinkle with about 1/2 cup mozzarella followed by half of the meat ingredients.

7. Continue layering with cheese and meat.

8. Bake until golden brown and bubbly (about 25 minutes).

9. Let it sit for 3–5 minutes before slicing.

Nutrition:

- **Calories:** 542
- **Carbs:** 24g
- **Fat:** 4g
- **Protein:** 32g
- **Sodium:** 1685mg

43. Olive Garden Classic Pepperoni

Preparation time: 15 minutes.

Cooking time: 12–15 minutes.

Servings: 8

Ingredients:

- 1 thin-crust pizza dough, or any dough of choice
- ½ -3/4 basic pizza or marinara sauce
- 2 cups mozzarella, freshly shredded

Directions:

1. Preheat the oven to 500°F.
2. Spread sauce over the crust.
3. Sprinkle with cheese.
4. Top with mozzarella.
5. Bake until golden and bubbly (about 12–15 minutes).

Nutrition:

- **Calories:** 276
- **Carbs:** 25g
- **Fat:** 14g
- **Protein:** 12g ; **Sodium:** 656mg

44. Olive Garden Meat with Bell Pepper & Mushrooms

Preparation time: 15 minutes.

Cooking time: 30 minutes.

Servings: 8

Ingredients:

- 1 pizza crust of choice
- ½ -3/4 cup marinara sauce
- 2 cups mozzarella, freshly shredded
- 1(1/2)-2 pounds seasoned beef or pork
- 16-24 pieces pepperoni
- 1 cup mushrooms, sliced thinly
- 1 medium green bell pepper, sliced thinly
- 1 red onion, sliced

Seasoned meat topping:

- 2 pounds ground lean beef or pork (or a combination)
- 1 teaspoon ground black pepper
- 1 teaspoon dried parsley
- 1 teaspoon oregano
- 1 teaspoon dried basil
- 1/2 teaspoon garlic powder
- 1/2 teaspoon onion powder
- 1/8 teaspoon chilli flakes
- 1/2 teaspoon paprika
- 2 teaspoons salt

Directions:

1. Preheat the oven to 425ªF.
2. Prepare the meat topping. Mix all the ingredients together well and sauté over medium heat until well-browned (about 10 minutes). Remove from heat and let cool.
3. Spread sauce over crust and sprinkle with cheese.
4. Top with seasoned meat, pepperoni, mushrooms, bell pepper, and onion.
5. Bake until golden brown (about 20 minutes).

Nutrition:

- **Calories:** 496
- **Carbs:** 27g
- **Fat:** 30g
- **Protein:** 27g
- **Sodium:** 1096mg

45. Chipotle's Refried Beans

Preparation Time: 5 minutes

Cooking Time: 5 minutes

Servings: 6

Ingredients:

- 1-pound dried pinto beans
- 6 cups warm water
- ½ cup bacon fat
- 2 teaspoons salt
- 1 teaspoon cumin
- ½ teaspoon black pepper
- ½ teaspoon cayenne pepper

Directions:

Rinse and drain the pinto beans. Check them over and remove any stones. Place the beans in a Dutch oven and add the water. Bring the pot to a boil, reduce the heat, and simmer for 2 hours, stirring frequently.

When the beans are tender, reserve ½ cup of the boiling water and drain the rest. Heat the bacon fat in a large, deep skillet. Add the beans 1 cup at a time, mashing and stirring as you go. Add the spices and some of the cooking liquid if the beans are too dry.

Nutrition:

- **Calories:** 100
- **Carbs:** 18g
- **Fat:** 1g
- **Protein:** 6g

46. Easy Copycat Monterey's Little Mexico Queso

Preparation Time: 15 minutes

Cooking Time: 10 minutes

Servings: 6

Ingredients:

- 1/2 cup of chopped yellow onion
- 1/2 cup of finely chopped celery
- 2 large green peppers such as Anaheim or Hatch, finely diced
- 2 tablespoons of butter
- 1 pound of American cheese
- 1/3 cup milk

Directions:

The real mystery of flavored cheese is to fry vegetables till they're almost wholly cooked when you begin adding a little crunch to your American cheese.

Place the chopped onion, thinly sliced celery, and diced pepper in a casserole over medium warmness, upload tablespoons of oil, and cook until the onion is transparent. Put in a medium bowl, American cheese, sautéed onions, and milk. Heat until low or medium warmness melts the cheese.

Nutrition:

- **Calories:** 226
- **Carbohydrates:** 4g
- **Protein:** 9g
- **Fat:** 18g

47. Fried Keto Cheese with Mushrooms

Preparation Time: 10 minutes

Cooking Time: 20 minutes

Servings: 4

Ingredients:

- 300 g mushrooms
- 300 g halloumi cheese
- 75 g butter 10 green olives
- salt and ground black pepper
- 125 ml mayonnaise (optional)

Directions:

Rinse and trim the mushrooms and chop or slice them. Heat the right quantity of butter in a pan in which they match and halloumi cheese and mushrooms.

Fry the mushrooms over medium heat for 3-5 minutes till golden brown. If vital, add extra butter and fry the halloumi cheese for a few minutes on every side. Stir the mushrooms occasionally.

Lower the warmness towards the end. Serve with olives.

Nutrition:

- **calories:** 169
- **total fats:** 17g
- **protein:** 10g

48. Mozzarella Cheese Sticks Recipe

Preparation Time: 5 minutes

Cooking Time: 5 minutes

Servings: 10

Ingredients:

- ¼ cup flour
- 1 cup breadcrumbs
- 2 eggs
- 1 tablespoon milk
- 500 g mozzarella cheese
- 1 cup of vegetable oil
- 1 cup marinara sauce

Directions:

Gather all the elements of mozzarella cheese sticks then mix eggs and milk together in a medium bowl. Cut the mozzarella into sticks 2 x 2 cm thick.

Cover each mozzarella cane with flour. Then dip them inside the egg and then within the breadcrumbs.

Dip the mozzarella sticks lower back into the egg and skip them in breadcrumbs.

Take to the freezer earlier than frying. Heat the oil within the pan and prepare dinner the mozzarella cheese sticks for approximately a minute on every aspect or until well browned.

Drain the cheese sticks on paper napkins and serve with marinara sauce or pizza sauce.

Nutrition:

- **calories:** 168
- **total fats:** 19g
- **protein:** 12g

49. Copycat Mac and Cheese with Smoked Gouda Cheese and Pumpkin

Preparation Time: 5 minutes

Cooking Time: 15 minutes

Servings: 6

Ingredients:

- 1 1/2 tbsp olive oil
- 120 grams of fresh baguette torn into small pieces
- 2 teaspoons fresh thyme leaves
- 1/4 cup grated Parmesan
- 450 grams of spiral pasta (or penne)
- 4 tablespoons salted butter
- 4 tablespoons of flour
- 3 cups room temp milk
- 1 cup canned pumpkin puree
- 2 cups smoked and chopped gouda cheese
- 2 cups cut sharp cheddar
- 21/2Kosher Salt

Directions:

Preheat oven to 190°C. Grease a large pan with nonstick cooking spray.

In a massive bowl, combine the cornbread, olive oil, thyme, and ½ tsp kosher Salt. Put in greased pan and bake till golden brown (12 to 15 minutes). Remove from oven, incorporate grated Parmesan, and set aside.

In a large pan of boiling salted water, cook the pasta al dente in line with package deal directions. Drain the water and set aside the pasta.

Melt butter in a pan over medium heat. Incorporate the flour and cook dinner, continually stirring, till the aggregate starts to thicken (about one to mins).

Gradually include the milk, continually mixing until its paperwork a lightly thickened sauce (five to six minutes). Add the mashed pumpkin and two teaspoons of kosher salt. Beat till included adequately into the sauce. Lower the warmth and location, the gouda and cheddar cheeses, mixing nicely until melted.

Incorporate the cooked pasta into the sauce. Transfer the whole lot to a prepared baking sheet. Sprinkle with toasted breadcrumbs. Put in oven and let till golden and blistered (about 20 mins). Serve immediately.

Nutrition:

- **calories:** 159
- **total fats:** 15g
- **protein:** 12g

50. Baked Buffalo Meatballs

Preparation Time: 5 minutes

Cooking Time: 20 minutes

Servings: 4

Ingredients:

- 350 gram of ground chicken meat
- 1 clove of minced garlic
- 1/4 cup of ground bread
- 2 tablespoons grated parmesan
- 2 teaspoons fresh celery leaves
- 1 egg
- 1/4 cup flour
- salt and pepper to taste
- 1/2 cup botanica sauce (Valentina or buffalo botanica)
- 2 tablespoons melted butter
- 1 tablespoon apple cider
- vinegar
- garlic powder and celery salt to taste for blue cheese dressing
- 1/3 cup of mayonnaise
- 1/3 cup sour cream
- 1 tablespoon lemon juice
- 1/4 cup blue cheese salt and pepper to taste

Directions:

Preheat the oven to 190°C Mix the chook with the garlic, the ground bread, the Parmesan, the celery, the egg, and the flour. Form balls together with your arms and region them on a tray with foil; bake for 18 mins.

Mix the botanica sauce with the melted butter and season with garlic powder and celery salt, bathe on this sauce every meatball as quickly as they go away from the oven.

To make the dressing, blend the cream, mayonnaise, lemon, and half of the blue cheese; upload the relaxation of the crumbled cheese and season to taste. Serve the meatballs with chopsticks observed via blue cheese dressing.

Nutrition:

- **calories:** 170
- **total fats:** 16g
- **protein:** 13g

Chapter 7: Chili's

51. Chili's Black Bean

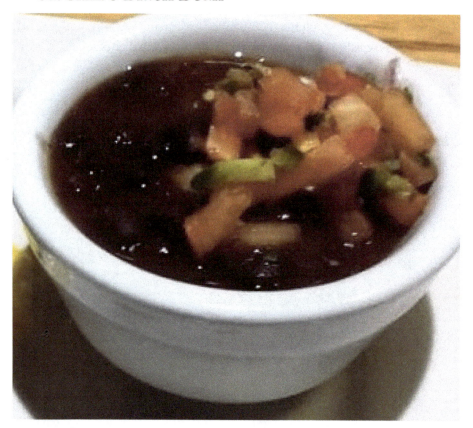

Preparation time: 5 minutes

Cooking time: 25 minutes

Servings: 6

Ingredients:

- 2 cans (15.5-ounces each) black beans
- ½ teaspoon sugar
- 1 teaspoon ground cumin
- 1 teaspoon chili powder
- ½ teaspoon garlic powder

- 2 tablespoons red onion, diced finely
- ½ teaspoon fresh cilantro, minced (optional)
- ½ cup water
- Salt and black pepper to taste
- Pico de Gallo and or sour cream for garnish (optional)

Directions:

Combine the beans, sugar, cumin, chili powder, garlic, onion, cilantro (if using), and water in a saucepan and mix well.

Over medium-low heat, let the bean mixture simmer for about 20-25 minutes. Season with salt and pepper to taste.

Remove the beans from heat and transfer them to serving bowls.

Garnish with Pico de Gallo and/or a dollop of sour cream, if desired.

Nutrition:

- **Calories:** 365
- **Fat:** 12g
- **Fiber:** 26
- **Carbs:** 21g
- **Protein:** 32g

52. Chili's Baby Back Ribs

Preparation time: 15 minutes

Cooking time: 3 hours

Servings: 4

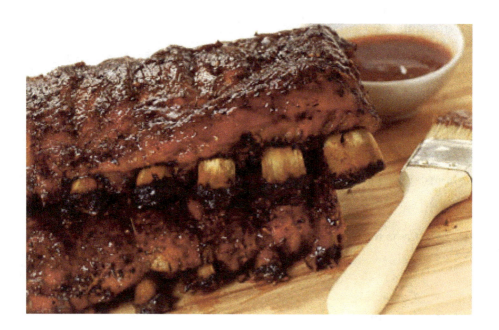

Ingredients:

Pork

- 4 racks baby-back pork ribs

Sauce

- 1 1/2 cups water
- 1 cup white vinegar
- 1/2 cup tomato paste
- 1 tablespoon yellow mustard
- 2/3 cup dark brown sugar packed

- 1 teaspoon hickory flavored liquid smoke
- 1 1/2 teaspoons salt
- 1/2 teaspoon onion powder
- 1/4 teaspoon garlic powder
- 1/4 teaspoon paprika

Directions:

1. Mix together all of the sauce ingredients and then bring to a boil.
2. When the sauce starts to boil, reduce it to a simmer. Continue simmering the mixture for 45 to 60 minutes, mixing occasionally. When the sauce is almost done, preheat the oven to 300 degrees F.
3. Choose a flat surface and lay some aluminum foil over it, enough to cover 1 rack of ribs. Place the ribs on top.
4. Remove the sauce from heat and start brushing it all over the ribs.
5. When the rack is completely covered, wrap it with the aluminum foil and place it on the baking pan with the opening of the foil facing upwards.
6. Repeat steps 3 to 5 for the remaining racks.
7. Bake the ribs for 2 1/2 hours.
8. When they are almost done baking, preheat your grill to medium heat.
9. Grill both sides of each rack for 4 to 8 minutes. When you are almost done grilling, brush some more sauce over each side and grill for a few more minutes. Make sure that the sauce doesn't burn.
10. Transfer the racks to a large plate and serve with extra sauce.

Nutrition:

Calories: 251

Carbs: 2g

Fat: 9.2g

Protein: 9.3g

53. Copycat Chili's Southwest Egg Rolls

Preparation Time: 5 minutes

Cooking Time: 15 minutes

Servings: 4

Ingredients:

- 8 oz chicken breast
- 1 teaspoon of olive oil vegetable oil is fine
- 1 tablespoon of olive oil vegetable oil is fine
- 1/4 cup chopped red bell pepper
- 1/4 cup chopped spring onions
- 1/2 cup frozen corn
- 1/2 cup canned black beans
- 1/4 cup frozen spinach
- 2 tsp of pickled jalapeno pepper
- 1 teaspoon of taco spice
- 3/4 cups of grated Monterey Jack cheese
- 8/7-inch flour tortillas
- 1/4 cup mashed fresh avocados (about half an avocado)

- 1 pack of Ranch Dressing Mix
- 1/2 cup milk
- 1/2 cup mayonnaise
- 2 tablespoons of chopped tomatoes
- 1 tablespoon of chopped onions

Directions:

Season with salt and black pepper to the fowl. Brush the fowl breast with olive oil. Grill on a grill with medium heat. Cook on each side for five to 7 mins. Cut the hen into tiny pieces. Set apart the fowl.

Sauté till tender red pepper. Refer to the aggregate of the green onion, rice, black beans, spinach, and pickled jalapenos. Attach the seasoning of the taco. Via the sun.

Place the tortillas in the same quantities of the filing, identical amounts of chicken, and pinnacle with cheese. Fold and roll-up on the ends of the tortilla. Make positive the tortillas are very tight to roll. To defend the pin with toothpicks.

We are growing enough vegetable oil in a big pot to cover the pan's backside through 4 inches. Heat up to 350°C. Deep fry the rolls of the eggs until golden brown. It ought to take seven to eight mins. When extracting golden from oil, growing it on a rack of wire.

Prepare a container of mayonnaise half-cup ranch dressing mix and buttermilk half of cup. Remove the aggregate 1/4 cup of mashed avocado. In a blender, pump the combination till the sauce is mixed.

Nutrition:

- **Calories:** 502
- **Carbohydrates:** 42g
- **Protein:** 19g
- **Fat:** 28g

54. Chili's Chicken Enchilada Soup

Preparation Time: 20 minutes

Cooking Time: 40 minutes

Servings: 8

Ingredients:

- 3 cooked chicken breast
- 1 1/2 tsp. garlic, minced
- 2 cans of chicken broth
- 1 cup corn tortilla mix
- 3 cups of water
- 1 cup mild enchilada sauce
- 15 ounces Velveeta cheese
- 1 tsp. salt
- 1/2 tsp. cumin
- 1 tsp. onion powder
- 1/2 tsp. chili powder

Directions:

In a large pot, add the garlic and sauté for 1-2 minutes.

Add broth to chicken.

Whisk together masa harina and 2 cups of water in a medium bowl until well mixed. Add masa to the pot.

Add the remaining water, enchilada sauce, Velveeta cheese, salt, cumin, onion powder, and chili powder. Take to simmer.

Attach the chicken cubed, raising oil, and simmer for half an hour.

Garnish with red tomatoes and tortilla.

Nutrition:

- **Calories:** 356
- **Fat:** 53.9 g
- **Carbs:** 25. 6 g
- **Protein:** 12.8 g ; **Sodium:** 454 mg

55. Cajun Chicken Pasta from Chili's

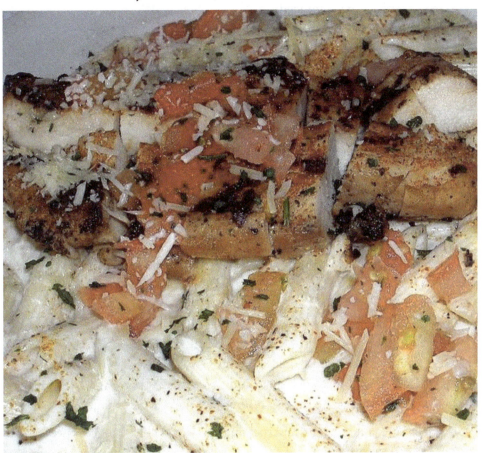

Preparation Time: 10 minutes

Cooking Time: 20 minutes

Servings: 4

Ingredients:

- 2 chicken breasts, boneless and skinless
- 1 tablespoon olive oil, divided
- 1 tablespoon Cajun seasoning
- 3 quarts' water
- ½ tablespoon salt
- 8 ounces penne pasta

- 2 tablespoons unsalted butter
- 3 garlic cloves, minced
- 1 cup heavy cream
- ½ teaspoon lemon zest
- ¼ cup Parmesan cheese, shredded
- Salt and black pepper, to taste
- 1 tablespoon oil
- 2 Roma tomatoes, diced
- 2 tablespoons parsley chopped

Directions:

Place chicken in a Ziploc bag. Add 1 tablespoon oil and Cajun seasoning. Using your hands, combine chicken and mixture until well-coated. Seal tightly and set aside to marinate.

Cook pasta in a pot filled with salt and boiling water. Follow package instructions. Drain and set aside.

In a skillet, heat butter over medium heat. Sauté garlic for 1 minute or until aromatic. Slowly add cream, followed by lemon zest. Cook for 1 minute, stirring continuously until fully blended. Toss in Parmesan cheese. Mix until sauce is a little thick, then add salt and pepper. Add pasta and combine until well-coated. Transfer onto a bowl and keep warm.

In a separate skillet, heat the remaining oil. Cook chicken over medium-high heat for about 5 minutes on each side or until fully cooked through. Transfer onto a chopping board and cut into thin strips.

Top pasta with chicken and sprinkle with tomatoes and parsley on top.

Serve.

Nutrition:

- **Calories:** 655
- **Total Fat:** 38 g
- **Carbs:** 47 g
- **Protein:** 31 g
- **Sodium:** 359 mg

© Copyright 2020 by _____ - All rights reserved.

The following Book is reproduced below with the goal of providing information that is as accurate and reliable as possible. Regardless, purchasing this Book can be seen as consent to the fact that both the publisher and the author of this book are in no way experts on the topics discussed within and that any recommendations or suggestions that are made herein are for entertainment purposes only. Professionals should be consulted as needed prior to undertaking any of the action endorsed herein.

This declaration is deemed fair and valid by both the American Bar Association and the Committee of Publishers Association and is legally binding throughout the United States.

Furthermore, the transmission, duplication, or reproduction of any of the following work including specific information will be considered an illegal act irrespective of if it is done electronically or in print. This extends to creating a secondary or tertiary copy of the work or a recorded copy and is only allowed with the express written consent from the Publisher. All additional right reserved.

The information in the following pages is broadly considered a truthful and accurate account of facts and as such, any inattention, use, or misuse of the information in question by the reader will render any resulting actions solely under their purview. There are no scenarios in which the publisher or the original author of this work can be in any fashion deemed liable for any hardship or damages that may befall them after undertaking information described herein.

Additionally, the information in the following pages is intended only for informational purposes and should thus be thought of as universal. As befitting its nature, it is presented without assurance regarding its prolonged validity or interim quality. Trademarks that are mentioned are done without written consent and can in no way be considered an endorsement from the trademark holder.

© Copyright 2020 by Luis Smith- All rights reserved.

The following Book is reproduced below with the goal of providing information that is as accurate and reliable as possible. Regardless, purchasing this Book can be seen as consent to the fact that both the publisher and the author of this book are in no way experts on the topics discussed within and that any recommendations or suggestions that are made herein are for entertainment purposes only. Professionals should be consulted as needed prior to undertaking any of the action endorsed herein.

This declaration is deemed fair and valid by both the American Bar Association and the Committee of Publishers Association and is legally binding throughout the United States.

Furthermore, the transmission, duplication, or reproduction of any of the following work including specific information will be considered an illegal act irrespective of if it is done electronically or in print. This extends to creating a secondary or tertiary copy of the work or a recorded copy and is only allowed with the express written consent from the Publisher. All additional right reserved.

The information in the following pages is broadly considered a truthful and accurate account of facts and as such, any inattention, use, or misuse of the information in question by the reader will render any resulting actions solely under their purview. There are no scenarios in which the publisher or the original author of this work can be in any fashion deemed liable for any hardship or damages that may befall them after undertaking information described herein.

Additionally, the information in the following pages is intended only for informational purposes and should thus be thought of as universal. As befitting its nature, it is presented without assurance regarding its prolonged validity or interim quality. Trademarks that are mentioned are done without written consent and can in no way be considered an endorsement from the trademark holder.

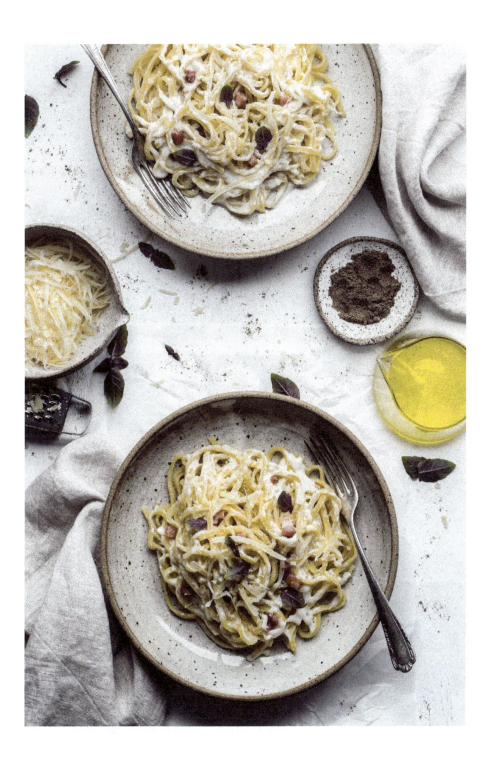

CPSIA information can be obtained
at www.ICGtesting.com
Printed in the USA
LVHW061320300321
682947LV00002B/30